WHO HANDBOOK FOR STANDARDIZED CANCER REGISTRIES

WORLD HEALTH ORGANIZATION

GENEVA

1976

WHO offset publications are intended to make generally available material that for economic, technical, or other reasons cannot be included in WHO's regular publications programme and would otherwise receive only limited distribution. They are usually reproduced by photo-offset from typescript, rather than by letterpress, and do not necessarily receive such detailed editorial revision as other WHO publications.

ISBN 92 4 170025 4

CONTENTS

                                                                    Page

Introduction   4

Aims of hospital-based cancer registries   6

Aims of population-based cancer registries   7

Functions of hospital-based cancer registries 7

Prerequisites for hospital-based cancer registries   7

Standardization of hospital-based and population-based cancer
    registries   9

Plan of the Handbook 10

Core data   11

Item 1: Identification of cancer registry   13

     2: Tumour registration number 14

         Identification of patient (items 3-10): explanatory
         note 15

     3: Personal identification number   16

     4: Name 17

     5: Sex   18

     6: Date of birth   19

     7: Birthplace 20

     8: Address   21

     9: Marital status 22

    10: Telephone number 23

    11: Age at first consultation or admission 24

    12: Date of first diagnosis of cancer   25

    13: Date of first consultation or admission to the
         reporting hospital for the cancer   26

    14: Hospital record number 27

    15: Previous diagnosis and treatment elsewhere 28

    16: Investigations relevant to the diagnosis of cancer
         as basis for planning the treatment   29

Item 17: Most valid basis of diagnosis of cancer 31

18: Primary site: topography (ICD) 33

19: Histological type: morphology (MOTNAC/ICD-O) 34

20: Multiple primaries 36

21: Clinical extent of disease before treatment at
reporting institution 37

22: Treatment at reporting institution 38

23: Subsequent description of extent of disease on the
basis of surgery or autopsy 39

24: Status at annual follow-up 40

25: Date of death 42

26: Cause of death (ICD) 43

27: Result of autopsy 44

28: Survival in months 45

Optional data 47

Item 51: Department of hospital 50

52: Nationality 51

Items 53-56: explanatory note 52

53: Religion 53

54: Ethnic group 54

55: Occupation 55

56: Industry 56

57: Reason for presentation of patient 57

58: Lymphoma (including Hodgkin's disease) and
leukaemias 59

59: TNM system 61

60: Site(s) of distant metastases 62

61: Co-morbidity 64

62: Conditions affecting treatment 66

63: Reasons for non-curative treatment 68

Page

Item 64: Laterality 69

65: Surgery 70

66: Radiotherapy 72

67: Chemotherapy 74

68: Hormonal therapy 76

69: Other therapy 78

70: Summary of treatment delivered 79

71: Chronology of treatment 81

72: Disease status at discharge from hospital 82

73: Duration of hospitalization in days 83

74: Patient status (i) before and (ii) after first
       treatment, and at anniversaries 84

75: Additional causes of death (ICD) 86

76: Cancer entered on death certificate 87

Standardized punch card 88

Recommended format for core data (first card) 90

Recommended format for optional data (second card) 91

Acknowledgements 92

List of participants at the consultations on the
    standardization of cancer registries 92

INTRODUCTION

The World Health Organization has always emphasized the aim of coordinating national efforts in the field of cancer control. The need for a "common language" in order to perform this task is obviously essential. In furtherance of this aim a programme of standardization of cancer registries has been developed.

Some of the difficulties of international cancer control arise because of a lack of standardization. These difficulties include:

(1) Differences in pathological nomenclature of malignant diseases;

(2) Differences in classification of malignant diseases;

(3) Differences in cancer staging;

(4) Differences in evaluation and presentation of results.

WHO is committed to activities aimed at resolving the first two differences enumerated, and the International Union Against Cancer (UICC) and the American Joint Committee for Cancer Staging and Results Reporting (AJC) are involved in overcoming the third; it was felt that a further step to help cancer control activities should be an attempt to standardize hospital cancer registries, which, of course, would use all those elements for which unification has already been achieved or is recommended (the International Classification of Diseases (ICD), the UICC's TNM[1] system for cancer staging, etc.).

In 1970, WHO undertook a survey of 26 hospital cancer registries from which it was apparent that the variation between them was so great as to exclude the possibility of comparative studies.

Several main conclusions were drawn from the survey:

(1) The aim of hospital-based cancer registries was not well understood;

(2) In many instances the registries were created without sufficient study or understanding of the subject;

---

[1] T = the tumour; N = the regional lymph nodes; M = distant metastases.

(3)   The data registered and their formulation and terminology showed much variation - for example, five registries did not use the ICD, and two did not collect any diagnostic information.

(4)   Many of the data collected were of doubtful importance and of doubtful accuracy.

As a result of the survey three consultations have been held at WHO headquarters to discuss this subject.[1]   At the first, held in November 1971, three main requirements were agreed upon:

(1)   The proposed registry system should be usable in any country, developed or developing;

(2)   The proposed registry system should be ready for immediate use.

(3)   It should overcome language barriers, using the same number for each item for comparative purposes.

The report[2] of this consultation summarized the objectives and some of the data requirements of hospital-based cancer registries.

At a second consultation a standard record card was designed and recommended for field trial.   It was divided into two sections: the first included core data, to be collected by all registries, and the second optional data.   Analyses of the results obtained from the field trial were discussed at the third consultation and the final standardized data format presented in this Handbook was produced.   It was realized at this third consultation that the core data to be used by hospital-based cancer registries must be equally acceptable by population-based cancer registries, on the grounds that many registries serve both clinical and epidemiological purposes.

---

[1] A list of participants appears at the end of this Handbook.

[2] Unpublished;   copies are available to persons officially or professionally interested on request to Cancer unit, WHO, Geneva, Switzerland.

AIMS OF HOSPITAL-BASED CANCER REGISTRIES

The aims of hospital-based cancer registries can be summarized as follows:

A.   From the viewpoint of the cancer institute, or specialized departments of hospitals:

   (1)   To facilitate the follow-up of all patients for clinical purposes;

   (2)   To provide data on survival of patients:
      (a)   for different cancer sites
      (b)   in relation to treatment methods and policies
      (c)   in relation to the natural history of cancer;

   (3)   To provide data on changes and trends in treatment methods with time;

   (4)   To give the total number of patients seen annually, categorized by site of cancer;

   (5)   To furnish exact figures of the demands made by cancer patients on the facilities, personnel and resources of the institution, including changes in those demands with time, so as to establish a better basis for planning.

B.   From the viewpoint of the general cancer care situation, to provide data and services such as:

   (6)   Number of cases diagnosed and/or treated in the hospital catchment area;

   (7)   Ratio between localized and advanced cases at time of diagnosis and the change in this ratio year by year;

   (8)   Information required by population-based cancer registries, if existing;

   (9)   To facilitate the exchange of information and the organization of collaborative studies with population-based cancer registries, where these exist, and with other hospital cancer registries at the national or international level;

   (10)   Information for international cancer data banking system(s), if established in future.

AIMS OF POPULATION-BASED CANCER REGISTRIES

In general, such registries measure the incidence of cancer in a particular area for epidemiological purposes, such as, for example, research into etiology or migrant studies.   Some registries combine both functions and may be termed "mixed".

It is, of course, the aim of a population-based cancer registry to record every case of malignant disease occurring in the population with which it is concerned, free of any incidental bias that might otherwise distort its description of the disease. A hospital-based cancer registry, on the other hand, may well present a substantially biased picture of the disease, perhaps because of its own constitution as a specialist hospital for the treatment of malignant disease (if that should be the case), or as a radiotherapy centre, or as one confined to a particular specialty, such as gynaecology or diseases of the chest.   It is important that such biases should be emphasized when reports are published.

FUNCTIONS OF HOSPITAL-BASED CANCER REGISTRIES

From the aims enumerated above, two broad areas of activity of hospital-based cancer registries may be distinguished:

(1)   "Internal activities" - the function of the registry within the hospital is to provide data to enable patient care and follow-up to be pursued efficiently and to be evaluated, and to provide better patient management, both directly and indirectly, through the education of physicians and other staff.

(2)   "External activities" - to enable comparisons of the data from the registry to be made either within the country or on an international basis.

Even in a sophisticated country problems often arise in the comparison of data, and the standardization programme has been developed in an attempt to resolve them.

PREREQUISITES FOR HOSPITAL-BASED CANCER REGISTRIES

The basic prerequisites for hospital-based cancer registries are:

(1)   A records department (if not in existence, it must be created);

(2)   A basic clinical data sheet or file for each individual patient;

(3)   Adequate staff to operate the registry;

(4)   Provision for the training of such staff;

(5)   An interested clinician, who, if not in charge of the registry, would be available for consultation;

(6)   Access to the advice of a pathologist.

Although there may seem to be a possibility of conflict with existing hospital records departments, this is, in general, not likely to be a problem.   When hospital-based cancer registries are established in a general hospital there are some advantages to their being separated administratively from the hospital records department, though associated closely with it, as such records departments tend to be overworked and understaffed.

There are some circumstances where a hospital-based cancer registry would serve a number of hospitals;   it might then be established in a building separate from any of the hospitals.

It is highly desirable for a hospital-based cancer registry that the people who are going to use it should want it;   otherwise there is little possibility that they will cooperate with it.   These people are usually clinicians, though sometimes the necessity for a hospital-based cancer registry is first appreciated by hospital administrators and only subsequently do clinicians come to perceive the need for and the value of the registry.   Although very often the basic reason for the registry is to improve patient management by providing data on follow-up, some registries have been able to fulfil many of the administrative needs which brought them into existence without undertaking follow-up at all.

One of the difficulties in some existing registries has been that no real provision has been made for trained personnel to operate the registry and provide reports for the participants and interested agencies.

It is recommended:

(1)   That adequate provision should be made for appropriate personnel to operate hospital-based cancer registries;

(2)   That adequate provision should be made for training programmes designed to serve the needs of staff of hospital-based cancer registries;

(3)   That adequate finance should be provided both for staff salaries and for training programmes, not only in the areas where hospital-based cancer registries exist but require upgrading, but also in the areas where such registries have been proposed but have not yet been established.

STANDARDIZATION OF HOSPITAL-BASED AND POPULATION-BASED CANCER REGISTRIES

Since many hospital-based registries feed data to population-based registries, and other registries are mixed in type (i.e., they serve both hospital-based and population-based functions), it is obvious that all registries must use the same basic guidelines and identification systems.

It is recommended, therefore, that the guidelines included in this Handbook should be regarded as a basic standard for all registries.   For the measurement of cancer incidence only, it would be possible to delete such items as 1, 7, 8, 9, 10, 11, 14, 15, 19, 20, 21, 22, 23, 24, 25, 26, 27, and 28.

To reiterate the need for standardization - cancer registries are the sources from which many programmes of analysis and reports draw their data.   Unless the basic data are collected and presented in an agreed and standard manner, according to a common set of definitions, such reports coming from different parts of the world cannot be validly compared, and thereby a potentially valuable contribution to medical research is nullified.   Many well-known publications depend essentially on the compatibility of data from different sources, and they include studies concerned primarily with comparisons within a country, such as the Third National Cancer Survey[1] or the End Results in Cancer series of reports[2] in the United States of America, as well as international presentations such as Cancer Incidence in Five Continents,[3] where the problems created by the present lack of uniformity of standards are acutely apparent.   It is therefore not only highly desirable but in fact essential if the value of cancer data collected from all parts of the world is to be fully utilized that the definitions used should be standardized.   The importance of coordination of national

---

[1] Cutler, S. J. Report on the Third National Cancer Survey, Seventh National Cancer Conference Proceedings, Philadelphia, Lippincott, 1973.

[2] National Cancer Institute, Department of Health, Education, and Welfare, Washington, DC.

[3] 2nd ed., Geneva, International Union against Cancer, 1975.

efforts in the field of cancer research was emphasized by the World
Health Assembly in May 1974 (resolution WHA28.85).   The Health
Assembly furthermore stressed the need for a "common language" in
the tactical tasks of integrating these efforts, and for
standardization in its expression.

PLAN OF THE HANDBOOK

This book is concerned with the minimum standards which should
be applied in each hospital-based cancer registry.   Basically these
minimum standards concern the identification of patients and the
description of the cancer, and together they constitute the mandatory
core data.   Additional items can be recorded in individual
registries depending on local circumstances, the interests of the
participating physicians and the availability of information.   These
constitute optional data, many of which are highly desirable.   Each
item of core and optional data begins on a new page.   Such
guidelines and definitions as are appropriate to that item are
included, and space is left for the insertion of local notes and
coding systems.   It is absolutely necessary that the definitions
given should always be used, otherwise the ideal of comparability
will be lost.   For some groups of items the same explanatory
information is given under each item.   This procedure has been
adopted both for the convenience of users of the Handbook and in the
interests of exactitude.

Core information contains 28 items.   In order to overcome
language barriers the order of numbering of each item is of great
importance (e.g., item 20 will mean in all different languages
"multiple primaries").   In order to permit future amendments, the
numbers 29-50 are reserved.   Therefore, the optional data commence
with the number 51 and for the same purpose reservation is made up
to 100;   at the present time only the numbers 51-76 are in use.

<u>CORE DATA</u>

CORE DATA

Item 1: Identification of cancer registry:

This item should be related to a geographically based code, with provisions for subdivisions within countries, which might also permit it to be linked with other information of a similar kind, such as that published in Cancer Incidence in Five Continents.

This number is required for international collaborative studies and will be allocated by WHO at a later stage when the standardization programme is fully established.

Item 2:   <u>Tumour registration number</u>:   Seven digits

     Five digits for the tumour sequence number plus two additional digits preceding or following the number, to denote the year of registration, would be adequate.

     A tumour registration number is an essential identification item for each individual tumour.   It is necessary to identify each tumour, as distinct from the patient.   The reason for this is that a patient may have more than one tumour.   It is also possible that a patient may attend more than one hospital, and thus have different hospital numbers, and for this reason the tumour number cannot be equivalent to the hospital record number (item 14).

     A convenient tumour numbering system would include the year of registration at the beginning of the number, e.g.:

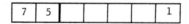

This would denote the first tumour to be recorded in 1975.

Identification of patient (items 3-10):   explanatory note

The next seven items constitute various features of patient identification.   Modes of identification vary from one country to another, and therefore it is not possible to prescribe exactly what should be used.   This group of items is intended to identify the patient unambiguously for two main purposes, first to minimize the likelihood of confusing him with any other patient, and second to facilitate the tracing of his progress when obtaining follow-up data. It is not appropriate to label these items separately as core data, but it is necessary to specify that, as a group, they should serve to identify the patient uniquely, and that in this sense they constitute an item of core data.   Date of birth is one of the most valuable items of personal identification, and if available should always be recorded.   If it is not available, then the age at first consultation or admission (when these dates were also specified) could count as the item of core data.   Whenever possible, both date of birth and age at first consultation or admission should be recorded in the core data.

Item 3: <u>Personal identification number</u>: Fifteen digits

  Many countries use a personal identification number which is unique to the individual concerned. It may also include other personal information, such as date of birth. The definition of this number is left to the registry itself. Some countries have no such number; others have more than one. If a suitable number is not available for virtually all patients, then it is probably better <u>not</u> to record it, and to depend on other means of patient identification.

Item 4: <u>Name</u>:

In some countries names can be valuable means of
identification. In other countries naming systems may create
serious confusion if used to establish identity. Therefore
the system of names should be standardized for each registry.
In some cases several standardized methods of naming may be
required. Most registries will need to record multiple names
(which would allow for changes - for example, on marriage) and
to cross-index them. When a patient has more than one entry
in the name file, it should be noted that there will,
nevertheless, be only one tumour registration number for that
patient, unless he has more than one tumour.

Item 5: <u>Sex</u>: One digit

> Subdivisions:

1 = Male

2 = Female

9 = Unspecified

> This item should always be coded.

Item 6: <u>Date of birth</u>: Six digits

     This should be recorded in <u>clearly labelled</u> boxes, such as in the form shown below:

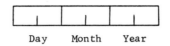

    Day   Month   Year

     Even when the date of birth forms part of a number listed in item 3 it should be listed here also.

     The <u>day</u> of birth is important identification information in those countries where some names are very common - e.g., there may be many people named John Smith but not many who were born on the 1st day of February 1934.

     For purposes of international collaboration it is necessary to convert any local dating systems to the standard system as used, for instance, by United Nations organizations. For comparative studies the order of day, month, year will be used. If day and month of birth are not available, at least the year of birth should be recorded.

Item 7:   <u>Birthplace</u>:

Whenever possible the precise birthplace in the country
or region of origin should be recorded.

This item is recorded for two purposes: (1) it may be
used to assist in identification;   (2) it may help to indicate
ethnic or cultural factors and as such may be important in
migrant studies.   For use in the latter way, a suitable code
would have to be designed by the individual registry as
optional data, otherwise this item would not normally be coded.

Item 8: <u>Address</u>:

This item is included here as part of the patient's
identification and should thus be the patient's usual residence.

It is generally regarded as desirable for every cancer
patient to be physically examined at least once each year.
The follow-up anniversary date (item 13) is often a convenient
time for this to be done. A number of other addresses may be
required in order to be able to contact the patient for
follow-up purposes. Examples might be the addresses of a near
relative, a near neighbour, the local doctor, or a person of
influence or authority who may assist with patient contact.
These addresses may be kept separately - e.g., in a special
follow-up file or in the hospital record.

Item 9: <u>Marital status</u>:

     The form in which this item of personal identification is recorded should be left to the individual registry.

     This item may provide an aid to identification in those countries where names are changed as a result of marriage. It is also relevant to certain sites of cancer, in particular of the reproductive system.

Item 10:   Telephone number:

The patient's telephone number may be of use in helping to establish identification, as well as in providing contact facilities.   If the patient has moved, it may be possible to trace his new address through the telephone company (especially for follow-up purposes).

Item 11:   <u>Age at first consultation or admission</u>:   Two digits

Subdivisions:

00   = Less than 1 year of age

01 - 97 = Age 1 - 97 (completed years)

98   = 98 or more

99   = Unspecified

This item should be coded and should be recorded in addition to item 6 for the reason that exact date of birth is sometimes difficult to obtain and also because it may be used as a check on item 6.

Item 12:   <u>Date of first diagnosis of cancer</u>:   Four digits (month and year)

The date of first diagnosis has been variously recorded in different registries, and even within a single registry, as "the date on which a physician first made a diagnosis of cancer", "the date on which a pathological diagnosis of cancer was made", or "the date of first admission to hospital where a diagnosis of cancer was made".   It is recommended that <u>the date of first diagnosis of cancer by a physician</u>, even if not confirmed histologically until later, or never confirmed histologically, is the one that should be used in standardized registries.   It is important for this date to be recorded if available, as it can be used as a measure of delay between the first diagnosis of cancer by a physician and definitive treatment of the disease.

As an example, a general practitioner feels a lump in a patient's breast and makes a diagnosis of possible cancer. The patient is referred to a hospital where the diagnosis is confirmed.   The date of diagnosis to be recorded is the date of the general practitioner's diagnosis.   If the hospital does not confirm the diagnosis, the case is not registered.

Item 13: <u>Date of first consultation or admission to the reporting</u>
<u>hospital for the cancer</u>: Four digits (month and year)

This date is the most consistently available item of
information throughout the world.   For this reason it has been
chosen as both the <u>anniversary date</u> for follow-up purposes and
the <u>date of occurrence</u> for measuring incidence.   For the latter
purpose it can only be used if the hospital in question is the
first one consulted (see also item 15).

Item 14: <u>Hospital record number</u>:

This item should always be recorded in order to facilitate reference back to hospital records for additional information not included in the cancer registry - e.g., what percentage of breast cancer patients had received treatment with <u>Rauwolfia</u> derivatives.

However, it is not recommended to include this item on the computer punch card.

Item 15:   <u>Previous diagnosis and treatment elsewhere</u>:   One digit

Subdivisions:

1 = No

2 = Diagnosed by physician only, but not treated

3 = Diagnosed in other institution, but not treated

4 = Diagnosed in other institution, and treated

9 = Unknown

This item refers only to previous treatment for the particular tumour being registered. It should always be coded. It is frequently necessary to exclude previously treated patients from analyses because of lack of information about details of previous treatment.

Item 16: Investigations relevant to the diagnosis of cancer as basis for planning the treatment: Three digits

Subdivisions:

First digit

1 = Purely clinical

2 = Laboratory methods

3 = 1 + 2

4 = Isotopes or X-rays

5 = 1 + 4

6 = 2 + 4

7 = 1 + 2 + 4

8 = None of these

9 = Unknown

Second digit

1 = Endoscopy

2 = Exploratory surgery

3 = 1 + 2

4 = Cytology and/or haematology

5 = 1 + 4

6 = 2 + 4

7 = 1 + 2 + 4

8 = None of these

9 = Unknown

Third digit

1 = Histology of metastatic tumour

2 = Histology of primary tumour

3 = 1 + 2

4 = Other (specify)

5 = 1 + 4

6 = 2 + 4

7 = 1 + 2 + 4

8 = None of these

9 = Unknown

Example: If the diagnosis has been based on a full <u>clinical examination</u>, <u>radiography</u> and <u>haematology</u>, the coding would be

| 5 | 4 | 8 |

     This item of information will sometimes be used to assess the quality of diagnosis before treatment - e.g., to discover what proportion of lung cancers have been confirmed histologically.   It may also be used to record recently introduced examinations in order to assess their value at a later stage - e.g., lymphangiography in relation to the management of lymphoma.   If such an item is recorded, in due course it will be possible to analyse the survival patterns of patients managed by this technique in comparison with those cases where it was not used.   This item of information must not be updated after the treatment has been initiated.

Item 17:   <u>Most valid basis of diagnosis of cancer</u>:   One digit

Subdivisions:

<u>Non-microscopic</u>

1 = Clinical only

2 = Clinical investigations (e.g., X-ray, isotopes, endoscopy, angiography, EEG)

3 = Exploratory surgery or autopsy but without histology

4 = Specific biochemical and/or immunological tests

<u>Microscopic</u>

5 = Cytology or haematology

6 = Histology of metastasis

7 = Histology of primary

8 = Autopsy with concurrent or previous histology

9 = Unknown

The recording system should be such that the nine categories listed above can be registered as core data.   This item of information will sometimes be used to assess the quality of diagnosis - e.g., to discover what proportion of lung cancers have been confirmed histologically.   It may be used to record recently introduced examinations in order to assess their value at a later stage - e.g., lymphangiography in relation to the management of lymphoma.   If such an item is recorded, in due course it will be possible to analyse the survival patterns of patients managed by this technique in comparison with those cases where it was not used.

When more than one of the above bases of diagnosis exist, code the one which was most indicative of the cancer.   The reason for this procedure is to indicate the strength or accuracy of the diagnosis of cancer at the time that treatment was planned and the item must be altered or updated in the light of information obtained after the patient's discharge from hospital (e.g., by the results of a subsequent autopsy).

Item 18:   <u>Primary site: topography (ICD)</u>:   Four digits

This coding should be taken from the current revision of the ICD.

Item 19: <u>Histological type: morphology</u> (MOTNAC/ICD-O): Five digits

Five digits have been provided for this item because that is what will be required for the revised version of MOTNAC, proposed for use in the forthcoming International Classification of Diseases for Oncology (ICD-O). Until ICD-O is introduced, however, only four digits will be required. MOTNAC (Manual of Tumour Nomenclature and Coding), published by the American Cancer Society, is the section of SNOP (Systematized Nomenclature of Pathology) which deals with tumours.

It is suggested that the present 4-digit form of MOTNAC coding be recorded as:

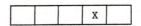

i.e., the fourth column should not be used, or as indicated the letter X should be placed in it. If this is done, the subsequent recording of the 5-digit form of ICD-O will be comparable with it, and will make use of the vacant space in the fourth column.

In developing the morphology section of ICD-O, a particular effort was made to include all the histological terms for neoplasms in the International Histological Classification of Tumours, published by WHO. These histological classifications are the result of a major international effort to develop criteria for the histological <u>definition</u>, <u>nomenclature</u>, and <u>classification</u> of neoplasms.

Item 20:   __Multiple primaries__: One digit

     Subdivisions:

1 = No

2 = Yes

3 = Doubtful

9 = Unspecified

     This item should be coded 2 (yes) when the physician in charge of the case is of the opinion that the patient has more than one separate or distinct tumour.   It is often not possible to be certain whether the tumours are multi-focal or separate. Subdivision 3 (doubtful) is therefore provided in order to differentiate on the record between clear-cut multiple primaries and those situations where there is doubt.   The former may be analysed in a routine fashion, but the latter may require a special investigation.   Some registries may wish to record only the number of multiple primaries as optional data.

     Whenever a further primary develops the initial card should always be altered and a new registration card should be completed for each additional primary.

Item 21: <u>Clinical extent of disease before treatment at reporting institution</u>: One digit

Subdivisions:

1 = In situ

2 = Localized

3 = Direct extension

4 = Regional lymph node involvement

5 = Direct extension with regional lymph node involvement

6 = Distant metastases

8 = Not applicable (i.e., lymphomas, see optional data item 58)

9 = Unknown

This item should reflect the opinion of the doctor in charge of the case except where a pathological report is available indicating carcinoma in situ. It should be recorded for **all** patients, whether or not previously treated elsewhere.

Item 22: <u>Treatment at reporting institution</u>: One digit

Subdivisions:

0 = No treatment

1 = Surgery

2 = Radiotherapy

3 = 1 + 2

4 = Chemotherapy

5 = 1 + 4

6 = 2 + 4

7 = 1 + 2 + 4

8 = Other therapy - specify

9 = Unknown

Where there has been no previous treatment elsewhere, this item will describe the definitive plan of treatment at the reporting institution. In some cases, part of this treatment may be subsequently delivered elsewhere. Where there has been previous treatment elsewhere, this item may be confined to describing treatment given at the reporting institution.

Item 23:   Subsequent description of extent of disease on the basis
           of surgery or autopsy: One digit

           Subdivisions:

1 = In situ

2 = Localized

3 = Direct extension

4 = Regional lymph node involvement

5 = Direct extension with regional lymph node involvement

6 = Distant metastases

8 = Not applicable (no surgery or autopsy)

9 = Unknown

        These codes are the same as for item 21 and should be used
in the same way to describe the extent of the disease on the
basis of surgery (including histology), or if the patient died
before treatment could be given and autopsy was performed.

Item 24:   Status at annual follow-up: Eight digits

Subdivisions:

1 = Alive, no evidence of cancer

2 = Alive, localized tumour

3 = Alive, direct extension or local involvement

4 = Alive, distant metastases

5 = Alive, subsequent primary discovered or first primary
    discovered when previously unknown

6 = Alive, nothing further specified

7 = No follow-up

8 = Dead

9 = Unknown

The information recorded here should wherever possible be obtained from the doctor in charge of the case.   With eight digits, provision is made for 1, 2, 3, 4, 5, 7, 10 and 15 years of survival.

Example: If the patient was followed up for the first three consecutive years with no evidence of tumour and only in the fourth year distant metastases appeared;   in the fifth year no follow-up was made, nor in the sixth, but in the seventh year the patient was reported dead, the coding would be:

1	1	1	4	7	8		
1	2	3	4	5	7	10	15

years of survival

Note that each box is allocated to one of the years of follow-up as indicated, and should be filled in, beginning from the left side.

Item 25:   <u>Date of death</u>:   Four digits (month and year)

Although it is only necessary to record the month and
year of death for core information, the exact date, including
day of month, should be written on the coding form because it
is often useful for tracing death certificates and other
information relating to the individual.

Item 26: <u>Cause of death (ICD)</u>: Four digits

This should be the underlying cause as defined in the ICD (see eighth revision, page 415, English edition).

Item 27: <u>Result of autopsy</u>: One digit

      Subdivisions:

1 = No autopsy

2 = No sign of residual tumour

3 = Primary site revised (give new ICD number)

4 = Morphological diagnosis revised (give new MOTNAC code)

5 = Diagnosis confirmed

6 = Case found at autopsy

7 = Diagnosis not confirmed (ICD code not confirmed)

8 = Autopsy performed, result unknown

9 = Unknown if autopsy performed

     In this item subdivision 2 indicates that the tumour had been completely removed or that the disease (e.g., leukaemia) was in remission. Subdivision 7 refers to cases where the autopsy examination suggests that the diagnosis of cancer was mistaken. It may be desirable to keep the punch card, but such a case should in general be excluded from incidence figures, whether relating to morbidity or mortality. (See also item 23.)

Item 28:   <u>Survival in months</u>:   Three digits

The date from which survival should be measured - the anniversary date (item 13) - should be the date of first hospital consultation or admission to the first hospital reporting the cancer.

OPTIONAL DATA

OPTIONAL DATA

Certain additional items of patient identification are included here rather than in the core data because they are not items of the highest priority.   Nonetheless, they do constitute a very important group of characteristics which may be associated with the incidence or the course of the disease. Since they distinguish subgroups of the population the data they provide may be used to give some indication of the extent of the differences in risk between such groups, even though it may not be feasible to relate them in the form of rates to their numbers in the whole population.

Item 52-56 are specifically aimed at distinguishing subgroups that may be of importance in special investigations either of incidence or of prognosis.

There is no reason why additional optional data may not be recorded.   However, where any of the items described here is registered the definitions given must be adhered to or the data will lack comparability.

Item 51: <u>Department of hospital</u>: Two digits

     This item is chiefly of local interest. If it is to refer to the department undertaking main treatment a two-digit code should be sufficient. If it is to record each department concerned with the treatment of a patient more space would clearly be required.

Item 52: <u>Nationality</u>: Three digits

For most purposes nationality is equivalent to citizenship. No standard code is proposed at present.

Items 53-56: explanatory note

It should be appreciated that the inclusion of items 53-56
may result in the expensive accumulation of confusing data
unless specific codes are established for specific studies.
It is not suggested that such items should be recorded purely
routinely but that they should be periodically monitored as
required.

Item 53: <u>Religion</u>: One digit

   Religion may be associated with various dietary patterns.
When religions prohibit the use of alcohol, for instance, the
rates for such tumours as oesophageal and liver may be affected.
Development of an appropriate code is left to the individual
institute or registry.

Item 54: <u>Ethnic group</u>: One digit

Certain ethnic groups may show special susceptibilities
(e.g., stomach cancer in Japanese, nasopharyngeal tumours among
certain Chinese, breast cancer among Caucasians, and
chorioncarcinoma in Malaysians). In many countries
a difference in living habits may be of interest for cancer
incidence (e.g., in Iran between town and country people, and
in India between the different castes), and even language
differences in some countries may indicate ethnic differences.
Development of an appropriate code is left to the individual
institute or registry.

Item 55: <u>Occupation</u>: No standard code is proposed at present.

Item 56: <u>Industry</u>: No standard code is proposed at present.

Beta-naphthylamine and bladder cancer, vinyl chloride and haemangiosarcoma of the liver, and asbestos and lung tumours are a few examples of relationships between industrial employment and cancer.

Item 57: __Reason for presentation of patient:__   One digit

Subdivisions:

1 = Advice

2 = Screening

3 = Diagnosis

4 = Initial treatment

5 = Complementary treatment

6 = Secondary treatment

8 = Other reason - specify

9 = Unknown

Under subdivision 1 "Advice" should be included those patients who have observed symptoms or signs by chance and seek advice, as well as those advised by family or friends to see a doctor.

Subdivision 2 "Screening" implies a specific screening test or a regular self-examination (e.g., self-palpation of breast).

Subdivision 3 "Diagnosis" applies to patients referred for diagnosis by other practitioners or hospitals.

Subdivision 4 "Initial treatment" refers to the first definitive treatment as defined in item 22, except that treatment carried out in another institution will be specified as "complementary".

Subdivision 5 "Complementary treatment" may refer to radiotherapy following surgery undertaken at another institution.

Subdivision 6 "Secondary treatment" refers to a subsequent course of treatment undertaken, for instance, because of failure to control the disease by the course of initial treatment.

Item 58: Lymphoma (including Hodgkin's disease) and leukaemias:
One digit

Subdivisions (1-4 provided exclusively for the staging
of lymphomas):

Lymphomas:

1 = Stage I

2 = Stage II

3 = Stage III

4 = Stage IV

There is still much dispute about staging systems for the
lymphomas. However, it is suggested that registries wishing
to record a staging system should use that proposed in 1970 by
Rosenberg & Kaplan (California Medicine, 1970, 113, 23-28).

Leukaemias:

5 = Active

6 = In remission

7 = No data on extent available

For lymphomas and leukaemias:

8 = Not applicable

9 = Unknown

Item 59: **TNM system**: Four digits

     This is an important system of recording the clinical
extent of disease in a standardized manner. Four digits are
provided for it, in order to allow for the addition of "+" or
"-" to indicate histological determination of involvement of
the lymph nodes (N).

     It is not possible to register this item <u>unless the
recording of the TNM is made in the medical record at the time
of the clinical examination.</u> Site specific TNM booklets are
available from the UICC describing in full the use of the
system.

<pre>
      T   N   M   N±
    ┌───┬───┬───┬───┐   N- = 1
    │   │   │   │   │   N+ = 2
    └───┴───┴───┴───┘
</pre>

Item 60:   <u>Site(s) of distant metastases</u>:   Three digits

Subdivisions:

0 = None

1 = Distant lymph nodes

2 = Bone

3 = Liver

4 = Lung and/or pleura

5 = Brain

6 = Ovary

7 = Skin

8 = Other (specify), or (3rd digit) Widely disseminated

9 = Not known

Example 1:   Distant lymph nodes involved

1	0	0

Example 2:   Metastases in bone and in brain

2	5	0

Example 3:   Bone, liver, brain

2	3	5

Example 4:   Carcinomatosis

		8

This item provides important and valuable information, and the recording should be as complete as possible.   Provision is made for recording, after the conclusion of treatment, up to three separate sites of distant metastases.   If there are more than three this should be recorded as "widely disseminated" by coding 8 in the third digit.

Item 61:   <u>Co-morbidity</u>:   One digit

      Subdivisions:

1 = No

2 = Yes: specify ICD numbers

    Most patients have some co-morbidity, and it is therefore sensible practice for a registry to create a special list of diseases which will be registered under this heading.   Three specific types of disease may be important:

      (1)   Precancerous conditions - e.g., polyposis coli or ulcerative colitis

      (2)   Conditions influencing the choice of treatment - e.g., cardiovascular conditions which may preclude surgery, or cirrhosis of the liver affecting response to a drug such as cyclophosphamide

      (3)   Conditions likely to affect the survival rate from cancers - e.g., diabetes or ischaemic heart disease.

    Under item 61 the ICD numbers for the specific conditions should be recorded.   Item 62 is included in order to allow punch card analysis of the broad categories listed therein as affecting treatment.

- 66/67 -

Item 62:   Conditions affecting treatment: One digit

Subdivisions:

0 = None

1 = Precancerous conditions or lesions

2 = Coexistent disease which may influence treatment

3 = 1 + 2

4 = Complications of the cancer or of the treatment

5 = 1 + 4

6 = 2 + 4

7 = 1 + 2 + 4

8 = Other - specify

9 = Unknown

Most patients have some co-morbidity, and it is therefore sensible practice for a registry to create a special list of diseases which will be registered under this heading.   Three specific types of disease may be important:

(1)   Precancerous conditions - e.g., polyposis coli or ulcerative colitis

(2)   Conditions influencing the choice of treatment - e.g., cardiovascular conditions which may preclude surgery, or cirrhosis of the liver affecting response to a drug such as cyclophosphamide

(3)   Conditions likely to affect the survival rate from cancers - e.g., diabetes or ischaemic heart disease.

Under item 61 the ICD numbers for the specific conditions should be recorded.   Item 62 is included in order to allow punch card analysis of the broad categories listed therein as affecting treatment.

Item 63:   <u>Reasons for non-curative treatment</u>:   One digit

       Subdivisions:

1 = Treatment given elsewhere

2 = Refused treatment

3 = Disease too advanced

4 = Poor general condition of patient

5 = Age

6 = Death

7 = Other - specify

8 = Not applicable

9 = Unknown

      Subdivision 8 "Not applicable" should be used where the treatment given is <u>curative</u>.

Item 64: Laterality: One digit

Subdivisions:

1 = Right

2 = Left

3 = Central

4 = Bilateral

5 = Multiple

8 = Not applicable (e.g., stomach)

9 = Unknown

This item is intended to refer to paired organs. Some registries may wish to establish a further optional item to register more detailed location within an organ - e.g., the breast.

Item 65: **Surgery**: One digit

Subdivisions:

1 = Symptomatic

2 = Palliative

3 = Curative (radical) - not completed

4 = Curative (radical) - completed

8 = Not applicable (no surgery)

9 = Unknown

The categories described under items 65-68 and 70 refer to the opinion of the doctor at the time of completion of definitive treatment - e.g., "curative, completed" should be recorded if the doctor thinks the operation has completely removed all trace of the tumour.   In some cases, time will show this opinion to be incorrect, but nevertheless it is important that the opinion on completion of treatment should be recorded and not changed because of subsequent events.

"Curative, not completed" refers to treatment undertaken with curative intent which was not completed because of operative complications or some other problems.

"Palliative treatment" is that given without expectation of cure but with expectation of prolonging or improving life.

"Symptomatic treatment" implies no expectation of prolonging life.

Item 66:   <u>Radiotherapy</u>:   One digit

      Subdivisions:

1 = Symptomatic

2 = Palliative

3 = Curative, not completed

4 = Curative, completed

8 = Not applicable (no radiotherapy)

9 = Unknown

    The categories described under items 65-68 and 70 refer to the opinion of the doctor at the time of completion of definitive treatment - e.g., "curative, completed" should be recorded if the doctor thinks the operation has completely removed all trace of the tumour.   In some cases, time will show this opinion to be incorrect, but nevertheless it is important that the opinion on completion of treatment should be recorded and not changed because of subsequent events.

    "Curative, not completed" refers to treatment undertaken with curative intent which was not completed because of operative complications or some other problems.

    "Palliative treatment" is that given without expectation of cure but with expectation of prolonging or improving life.

    "Symptomatic treatment" implies no expectation of prolonging life.

Item 67:   <u>Chemotherapy</u>:   One digit

Subdivisions:

1 = Symptomatic

2 = Palliative

3 = Curative, not completed

4 = Curative, completed

8 = Not applicable (no chemotherapy)

9 = Unknown

The categories described under items 65-68 and 70 refer to the opinion of the doctor at the time of completion of definitive treatment - e.g., "curative, completed" should be recorded if the doctor thinks the operation has completely removed all trace of the tumour.   In some cases, time will show this opinion to be incorrect, but nevertheless it is important that the opinion on completion of treatment should be recorded and not changed because of subsequent events.

"Curative, not completed" refers to treatment undertaken with curative intent which was not completed because of operative complications or some other problems.

"Palliative treatment" is that given without expectation of cure but with expectation of prolonging or improving life.

"Symptomatic treatment" implies no expectation of prolonging life.

Item 68:   <u>Hormonal therapy</u>:   One digit

Subdivisions:

1 = Withdrawal by surgery or radiotherapy

2 = Additive

3 = Antihormone therapy

8 = Not applicable (no hormonal therapy)

9 = Unknown

The categories described under items 65-68 and 70 refer to the opinion of the doctor at the time of completion of definitive treatment - e.g., "curative, completed" should be recorded if the doctor thinks the operation has completely removed all trace of the tumour.   In some cases, time will show this opinion to be incorrect, but nevertheless it is important that the opinion on completion of treatment should be recorded and not changed because of subsequent events.

"Curative, not completed" refers to treatment undertaken with curative intent which was not completed because of operative complications or some other problems.

"Palliative treatment" is that given without expectation of cure but with expectation of prolonging or improving life.

"Symptomatic treatment" implies no expectation of prolonging life.

Item 69: <u>Other therapy</u>: One digit

This item is provided for those registries wishing to
record other types of therapy - for instance, immunotherapy.
The subdivisions are optional, except that 8 should be "Not
applicable (no other therapy)", in conformity with items 65-68
and 70.

Item 70: **Summary of treatment delivered**: One digit

     Subdivisions:

1 = Symptomatic only

2 = Palliative

3 = Curative, not completed

4 = Curative, completed

5 = Uncertain

7 = Other

8 = Not applicable (no treatment)

9 = Unknown

    The categories described under items 65-68 and 70 refer to the opinion of the doctor at the time of completion of definitive treatment - e.g., "curative, completed" should be recorded if the doctor thinks the operation has completely removed all trace of the tumour. In some cases, time will show this opinion to be incorrect, but nevertheless it is important that the opinion on completion of treatment should be recorded and not changed because of subsequent events.

    "Curative, not completed" refers to treatment undertaken with curative intent which was not completed because of operative complications or some other problems.

    "Palliative treatment" is that given without expectation of cure but with expectation of prolonging or improving life.

    "Symptomatic treatment" implies no expectation of prolonging life.

Item 71:   Chronology of treatment: Six digits

This item gives the order in which the various component
types of treatment were given.   It allows for six successive
items of treatment (initial and subsequent treatments), and
each is to be entered in its appropriate position (starting
from the left) identified by a number according to the
following code:

1 = Surgery

2 = Radiotherapy

3 = Chemotherapy

4 = Hormonal therapy

8 = Other (specify)

9 = Unknown

Example: A patient was treated first by surgery, followed by
radiotherapy and chemotherapy.   Subsequently he received
a further course of radiotherapy, followed by chemotherapy.
This coding would be:

1	2	3	2	3	

Item 72: **Disease status at discharge from hospital**: One digit

    Subdivisions:

1 = No evidence of disease (cancer)

2 = Disease in regression

3 = Disease unchanged

4 = Disease in progression

8 = Died in hospital

9 = Unknown

    This item should record the opinion of the doctor in charge of the case at the time of discharge or at the end of hospitalization as defined in item 73.

Item 73: <u>Duration of hospitalization in days</u>: Three digits

     This item refers to the initial course of treatment given
in days.   It should include the time spent in hospital as
a result of treatment or direct complications but should not
include extension of hospital stay for social or other reasons.

Item 74: <u>Patient status (i) before and (ii) after first treatment,
and at anniversaries</u>: Ten digits

Subdivisions:

1 = Well and active

2 = Well, not active

3 = Some disability but active

4 = Some disability, not active

5 = Confined to bed

6 = Alive but no evidence of status

7 = No follow-up done

8 = Dead

9 = Unknown

This item reflects the quality of the patient's survival not the status of his tumour (item 28).

Two digits serve for the description of the patient's status before and after the first, or main and most important, treatment. The remaining eight digits refer to the patient's health status successively after 1, 2, 3, 4, 5, 7, 10 and 15 years of follow-up.

Example: A woman presenting with a breast tumour was, at the time of diagnosis, disabled but active. After treatment she was well and active. The first two digits would then be coded

as: | 3 | 1 |. For the first three years of follow-up her status remained unchanged ("well and active") but in the fourth year she became disabled and not active, and by the fifth year she was confined to bed. The coding for this case would be:

Before treat-ment	After treat-ment	Years of follow-up							
		1	2	3	4	5	7	10	15
3	1	1	1	1	4	5			

Item 75: <u>Additional causes of death (ICD)</u>: Twelve digits

Provision is made for up to three additional causes of death, each to be coded to four digits (ICD).

The underlying cause of death is recorded as core data in item 26. This item allows the other causes that may be mentioned on the death certificate to be recorded.

Item 76: <u>Cancer entered on death certificate</u>: One digit

Subdivisions:

1 = No

2 = Yes

9 = Unknown

This refers to any subsection of the international form of medical certificate of cause of death, including Section II (see ICD, eighth revision, page 416, English edition).

STANDARDIZED PUNCH CARD

Use of a standardized punch card will allow the transfer of data in collaborative studies to another institution or organization, such as WHO. Such a facility is the most convenient for many types of comparative studies including those of low incidence tumours.

For the convenience of registries using this Handbook, a standardized format for 80-column computer punch cards follows. This recommended format is a summary of the allocation of digits to each item of information. The starting position (column number) for each item should be printed on the tumour registration form, even if computer processing will not be locally available. Two computer cards are required for each registration form: one for core data (80 columns) and one for optional data (70 columns).[1]

For the purpose of collaborative studies, it will be convenient if the recommended format is followed exactly. It will be essential for any registry deviating from that format to provide a complete description of its own format. It is understood that some registries will not be able to code all the items of information. Even then, the recommended format may still be used, and the corresponding positions on the computer card left blank.

Ten columns are currently not used. They are available for recording additional items, if desired. If even more space were required, it would be preferable to introduce a third card, rather than alter the recommended format. If this is done, it should be linked with the preceding two cards by punching the first eleven columns (registry number and tumour registration number) with the same identification digits.

The punching of the computer cards should normally take place prior to placing the "completed" registration form in the registration master file. Obviously, some information will only

---

[1] For registries with access to equipment for the direct transfer of data to magnetic tape, it will of course be possible to create a single record length of 150 (80 + 70) positions, deleting the repetition of record identification (columns 1-7). The record length may be extended to include additional items, if desired, but the format for the first 150 positions should preferably not be altered.

become available at a later date (e.g., items concerning status at annual follow-up and death). Also, errors may occasionally be detected. Whenever a registration form is modified (corrected or updated), it is important that the modification should also be made to the corresponding computer record. In the case of 80-column punched cards, this may be done manually. In the case of magnetic tape systems, the responsible programmer will have to be notified, so that he can update the computer file.

RECOMMENDED FORMAT FOR CORE DATA (FIRST CARD)

		Number of digits	Positions
2	Tumour registration number	7	1- 7
3	Personal identification number	15	8-22
5	Sex	1	23
6	Date of birth	6	24-29
11	Age at first consultation or admission	2	30-31
12	Date of first diagnosis of cancer	4	32-35
13	Date of first consultation or admission to the reporting hospital	4	36-39
15	Previous diagnosis and treatment elsewhere	1	40
16	Investigations relevant to the diagnosis of cancer	3	41-43
17	Most valid basis of diagnosis of cancer	1	44
18	Primary site: topography (ICD)	4	45-48
19	Histological type: morphology (MOTNAC/ICD-0)	5	49-53
20	Multiple primaries	1	54
21	Clinical extent of disease before treatment at reporting institution	1	55
22	Treatment at reporting institution	1	56
23	Subsequent description of extent of disease on the basis of surgery or autopsy	1	57
24	Status at annual follow-up	8	58-65
25	Date of death	4	66-69
26	Cause of death (ICD)	4	70-73
27	Result of autopsy	1	74
28	Survival in months	3	75-77
29	Two columns free for locally important data	1	78
30	(To be allocated serial numbers beginning 101 or other higher number and not 29 and 30)	1	79
	Linkage (identifying the first card)		80

RECOMMENDED FORMAT FOR OPTIONAL DATA (SECOND CARD)

		Number of digits	Positions
2	Tumour registration number	7	1- 7
51	Department of hospital	2	8- 9
52	Nationality	3	10-12
53	Religion	1	13
54	Ethnic group	1	14
57	Reasons for presentation of patient	1	15
58	Lymphomas	1	16
59	TNM system	4	17-20
60	Site(s) of distant metastases	3	21-23
61	Co-morbidity	1	24
62	Conditions affecting treatment	1	25
63	Reasons for non-curative treatment	1	26
64	Laterality	1	27
65	Surgery	1	28
66	Radiotherapy	1	29
67	Chemotherapy	1	30
68	Hormonal therapy	1	31
69	Other therapy	1	32
70	Summary of treatment delivered	1	33
71	Chronology of treatment	6	34-39
72	Disease status at discharge	1	40
73	Duration of hospitalization in days	3	41-43
74	Patient status before treatment and at follow-ups	10	44-53
75	Additional causes of death (ICD)	12	54-65
76	Cancer entered on death certificate	1	66

ACKNOWLEDGEMENTS

WHO would like to express its gratitude to the participants in the series of consultations on the standardization of cancer registries (see following list) whose efforts made possible the production of this work.   Special thanks are due to Dr Nigel Gray and Dr J. A. H. Waterhouse, who acted as Chairman and Rapporteur respectively of the second and third consultations.   Dr A. Winkler, Medical Officer, Cancer unit, WHO, was the staff member most concerned with the organization and compilation of the Handbook.

LIST OF PARTICIPANTS AT THE CONSULTATIONS
ON THE STANDARDIZATION OF CANCER REGISTRIES

Dr A. L. Aboul-Nasr, Professor of Cancer Surgery, Cancer Registry for the Metropolitan Area of Cairo, Cairo, Egypt

Professor E. Anglesio, Director, Piemonte Cancer Registry, Turin, Italy

Dr D. P. Berezkin, Department of Organizational Research, the All-Union Centre for Study of End Results in Cancer, Research Institute of Oncology, Leningrad, USSR

Dr J. Berlie, National Institute of Health, Paris, France

Dr J. Galvez-Brandon, Chief, Epidemiology and Statistics Department, Cancer Registry of Metropolitan Lima, Lima, Peru

Dr V. N. Gerasimenko, Deputy Director, Institute of Experimental and Clinical Oncology of the USSR Academy of Medical Sciences, Moscow, USSR

Dr N. Gray, Director, Anti-Cancer Council of Victoria, East Melbourne, Australia (Chairman, second and third consultations)

Dr A. B. Miller, Assistant Executive Director, Cancer Institute of Canada, Toronto, Ont., Canada

Dr A. P. Mirra, Central Institute, A.C. Camargo Hospital, São Paulo, Brazil

Dr G. Mitrov, Director, Oncological Research Institute, Sofia, Bulgaria

Dr A. Modjtabai, Director, Taj Pahlavi Cancer Institute, Teheran, Iran

Dr N. Mourali, Director, National Cancer Institute, Tunis, Tunisia

Dr E. Pedersen, Director, Cancer Registry of Norway, Norwegian Radium Hospital, Oslo, Norway

Mr A. Ringel, Acting Associate Director of Health Care Systems, Regional Medical Programs, Rockville, MD, USA

Professor G. Riotton, Director, Centre of Cytology and Early Detection of Cancer, Geneva, Switzerland

Dr P. A. Salem, Assistant Professor of Medicine, Director of the Cancer Programme, American University Hospital, Beirut, Lebanon

Professor K. Shanmugaratnam, Professor of Pathology, Department of Pathology, University of Singapore, Singapore

Dr J. Staszewski, Oncological Institute, Gliwice, Poland

Dr V. Thurzo, Director, Cancer Research Institute, Bratislava, Czechoslovakia

Professor G. Wagner, Director, German Cancer Research Centre, Institute for Documentation, Information and Statistics, Heidelberg, Federal Republic of Germany

Dr J. A. H. Waterhouse, Director, Regional Cancer Registry, Queen Elizabeth Hospital, Birmingham, United Kingdom (Rapporteur, second and third consultations)

Professor C. Zippin, Professor of Epidemiology, General Tumour Registry, Cancer Research Institute, University of California, San Francisco, CA, USA

Short-term consultant

Dr W. P. D. Logan, Geneva, Switzerland

International Agency for Research on Cancer

Dr C. S. Muir, IARC, Lyons, France

International Union Against Cancer

Dr J. F. Delafresnaye, UICC, Geneva, Switzerland

Dr A. H. Sellers, Medical Statistician, Ontario Cancer Treatment and
Research Foundation, Toronto, Ont., Canada

Observers

Miss E. M. Brooke, University Institute of Social and Preventive
Medicine, Lausanne, Switzerland

Professor R. Flamant, Gustave-Roussy Institute, Villejuif,
Val-de-Marne, France

WHO Secretariat

Dr A. M. Garin, Chief, Cancer unit, Geneva

Dr H. E. Hansluwka, Chief, Dissemination of Statistical Information,
Geneva

Mr A. Thomas, Systems Analyst, Data Processing, Geneva

Dr A. Winkler, Medical Officer, Cancer unit, Geneva (Secretary)